THE BOOK OF
ENERGY

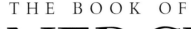

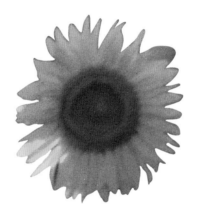

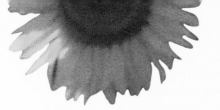

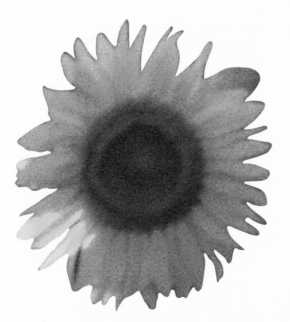

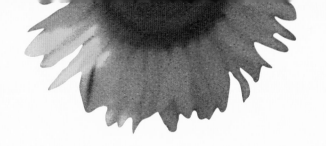
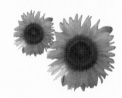

THE BOOK OF
ENERGY

Invigorating ways to
revitalize your life

CYNTHIA BLANCHE

TIME®
LIFE

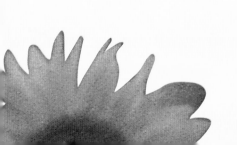

Contents

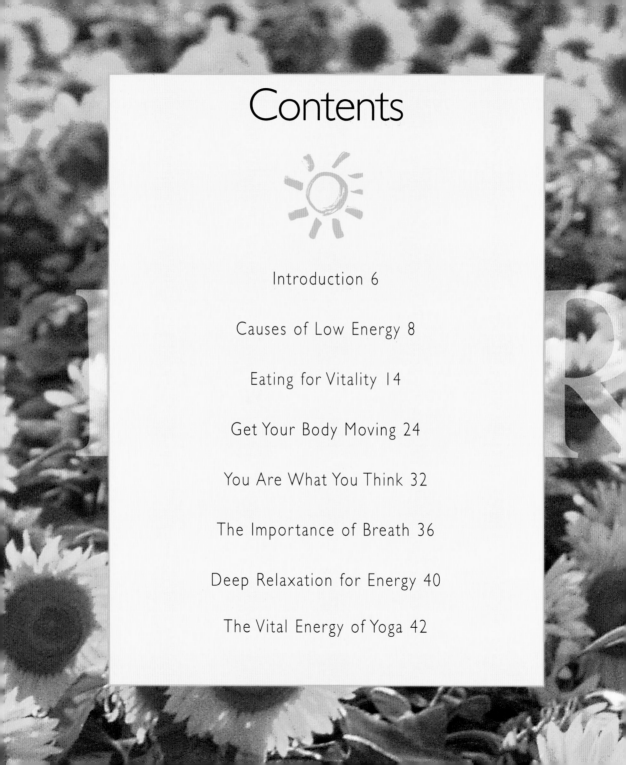

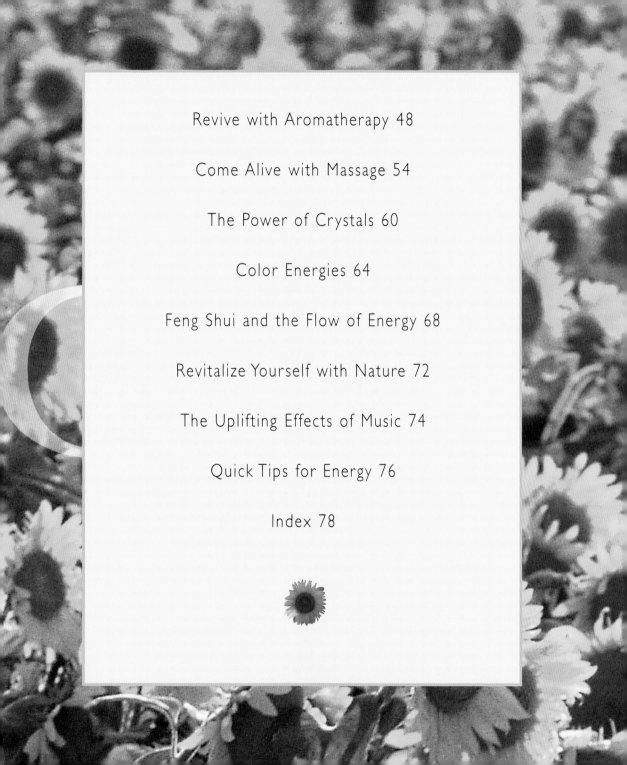

Introduction

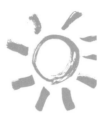

These days, many of us lack get up and go. With the best will in the world, we would often rather stay home and watch television than go to a show or visit some friends we haven't seen for some time. We tell ourselves that the theater is uncomfortable or that we'll visit our friends when the weather is warmer or cooler. But the fact is, we're just too tired to go out.

This book examines some of the causes of low energy, and offers some valuable advice to help you restore energy into your life. The cause of your lack of energy could be as simple as diet or long-term tension in your muscles, or you may need a little self-indulgence in baths and scents and meditation to remind yourself of who you are. There are medical problems that cause low energy levels, and many of these can be easily rectified after proper medical diagnosis. Even if your lack of energy comes from illness, or you are recovering from illness, this book will be of some benefit to you. All the information presented in these pages is designed to raise your energy levels in a safe and natural way.

Mental energy is also of great importance in undertaking any new venture, especially a challenging one. You might lose energy when confronted with a difficult problem or project, because of fear. The energy lost in panic could be put to better use, like in undertaking the challenge. This book offers tips on how to relax, harness, and then redirect that energy to a positive outcome.

It is true we are expected to work long hours. And some of us are, at the same time, parents whose children demand — and not unreasonably — our full attention. Eating well and exercise are essential for high energy, so is time to ourselves. Relaxation is just as important as nutrition and physical fitness if we are to experience lasting energy and its spin-off, enthusiasm for life. For the workaholic, a deep relaxation program can transform your excessive energy into a more evenly paced, productive pattern. Ideas and creative thinking, both necessary for the best productivity, require a relaxed mental space for contemplation and reflection. This book provides quick tips for relaxation and the renewal of energy while you are at work or at home.

Every person on the planet has to confront, at some time or another, emotionally draining situations. These are never easy to handle, but there are ways in which we can minimize the drain on our emotional energy, which in turn drains our physical and intellectual energies, and turn negative aspects into positive ones. Crystals, color and music, aromatherapy, meditation, and massage — this book provides tips and information on the ways you can utilize these gentle and beautiful techniques to help heal and restore your emotional well-being.

For increasing your energy levels or balancing them, the idea of this book is to help you rediscover the lightness of life, the joy of being alive. Every tip and technique in these pages can be done by you at home, either by yourself or with a partner, and with little cost involved. There is no need to go to expensive gyms to feel energized. All you really need is some floor space, a bed, a bath, a few inexpensive essential oils, and the desire to have control over your energy levels and your life.

Causes of Low Energy

When we suffer a persistent lack of energy we need to look for its cause. The next step is to undertake to do something about it to improve our quality of life.

In most cases, the reason for lack of energy is easily identified and easily fixed — this chapter outlines some of the most common causes.

There must be a physical, emotional, or mental basis for low energy. Sometimes the cause is easy to identify, in other cases a person might be so used to being low in energy that he or she has put it down to low metabolism or "it's just me, I was born that way."

Regardless of the cause of your low energy, you should find the information in this book beneficial, or, at the very least, comforting. A low energy level does not have to be your "lot in life."

Caution

Seek medical advice immediately if your tiredness comes on suddenly, and there is no obvious cause like overwork or unusual physical activity. It could be due to:

- Heart trouble • Blood disorders
- Lung diseases • Diabetes

Sleep Disturbances

Insomnia or disturbed sleep can be the result of worry about work or personal issues, or it can be the result of a bad mattress or pillow, the color of the room, or the way your bedroom furniture is placed.

Sleep will continue to evade you if you try to force it. If you are waking in the early hours of the morning, worrying about something, take one aspect of the problem and try to solve it, leaving the rest aside. Otherwise, read a book, get up and do something useful — but not stressful — and tell yourself that you are grateful for this time in the quiet and peace of the night. You will not be resentful and soon, a natural tiredness will overtake you and you will sleep.

Overwork

If you are in a high-stress career which demands a great deal of your time, you may find there seems to be nothing left for fun or just simple relaxation. If you work at this level, you are probably skimping on your diet, and eating fast foods, and lots of sugar to keep your energy up. You need to take stock of your day and how you are spending it. Organization is the key to doing everything you need to do without burning yourself out. There are ways to eat well without having to spend an hour or two at the stove each night. There are exercises and relaxation techniques you can do that take no time at all. All you need do is organize your time in advance, and set up your bathroom, your bedroom, your kitchen, and your office to maximize your time and energy.

Symptoms of Low Energy

- Unusual tiredness, even after 8 or 9 hours sleep

- Inability to summon enthusiasm

- Lack of interest in sex

- Poor concentration

- Apathy

Time for Yourself — Necessity, Not Luxury

If you are busy all the time, you are left with no time for yourself. Time for your thoughts, for catching up with who you are, is vital for emotional and physical well-being. If you deprive yourself, you will suffer stress, which will come out in ways that are hurtful not only to yourself, but to your children, partner, friends, and colleagues. The cost is not worth whatever rewards you think you're getting, especially since it doesn't take much to ensure you do have time for yourself.

Diet

Diet is the single most important aspect of building high energy. Without an adequate diet, you will continue to lose energy until you are unable to get up at all.

Fad diets do tremendous harm in this respect. Most fad diets for weight reduction are based on limiting carbohydrate intake and increasing proteins. Without carbohydrates you become tired, irritable and unable to get up and about.

You need to know what foods provide energy, and what foods rob you of energy. You also need to know when and how to eat to make the most of your energy supplies.

Medical Problems

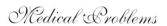

If you are recovering from a long illness you will have low energy levels. As well, there are over 200 illnesses — some serious, some relatively minor — that can cause low energy. If your energy levels are low and for no obvious reason — like overwork or too much physical activity — it is imperative you visit your medical practitioner for a complete physical check-up. Allergies, diabetes, lung disorders, thyroid problems, heart problems, cancer, blood disorders from mild anemia to leukemia, and menopause can all cause low energy.

Common Causes of Low Energy

• Physical or emotional stress • Sleep problems

• Poor nutrition or fad dieting

• Illness • Depression • Persistent low level pain

Emotional

When you feel good about yourself, you feel energized. When our emotions are negatively affected, by a relationship breakup, loss of a job, shyness, or depression, we lose confidence and the energy to make life exciting. We have no desire to go out and have a good time, we might even fear meeting new people.

Serious depression needs to be treated by a professional psychiatrist or psychotherapist. However, most cases of "not feeling great" can be treated by you at home. You need to restore your lack of confidence by getting to know yourself as a lovable human being. Pampering can be the way back to energy here, and there is nothing like aromatherapy and massage, with some exercise to enliven your sense of personal power, to begin the process. Visualizations and affirmations may also help restore your positive sense of self.

Chronic Fatigue or Chronic Fatigue Syndrome

Chronic fatigue is an unrelenting tiredness traceable to an inadequate diet, poor sleep patterns, emotional problems, doing too much, medical conditions (including following a virus), medications, smoking, and drinking. Sufferers of Chronic Fatigue Syndrome (CFS), on the other hand, experience extreme tiredness all the time, severe headaches, skin rashes, weakness in the arms and legs, and feel as though every muscle in the body is aching. People with this condition are usually unable to work or undertake normal day-to-day activities. To be categorized with CFS you must have experienced a disabling fatigue over a six month period at the very least, and the onset of your fatigue must be traceable to that time.

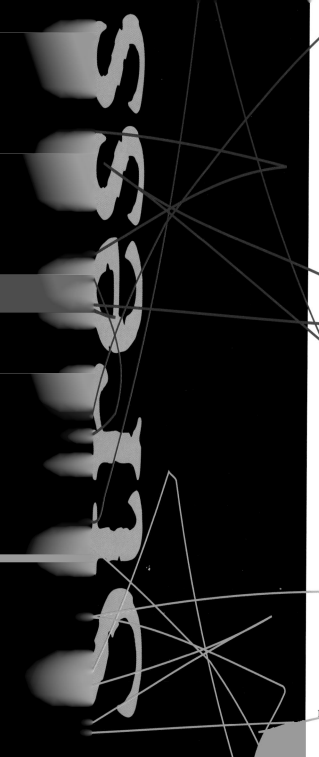

Stress

Stress can be caused by too much work. Repetitive or unsatisfying work, or not enough work, can also be stressful because of boredom and a possible effect on your self-esteem. It can be the result of too many demands being made on us all at the same time. For example, the mother of young children has to feed and dress her children, keep a constant eye on them, clean the house, do the shopping, do the laundry — and with a family all these activities are everyday events. The work begins early in the morning and doesn't end until late at night. Where is the time for some personal space? With a bit of organization and, hopefully, some support from partner, family, and friends, some can be made.

Stress at work can be the result of too much pressure or an insensitive boss or workmate. Good organization will save you time and energy, and will make you more efficient. The best way to deal with someone who doesn't behave well is not to let that person's attitude affect your self-esteem. Be friendly but distant, and never get caught up in any unnecessary dispute. You will be amazed at how quickly the bad attitude drops away when nothing is coming back to feed it!

Long-Term, Low-Level Pain

Many people suffer chronic, low-level pain for years without ever doing anything about it. Common low-level pain can be in your muscles, in your joints, in your teeth, in your neck. Pain uses a great deal of energy. It causes depression as well.

Go to your medical practitioner for advice. If he or she doesn't have an acceptable solution, at least get your doctor to isolate the problem, then try visiting a specialist in that field, e.g. a chiropractor or physiotherapist, a massage therapist, a dentist, or a dietitian.

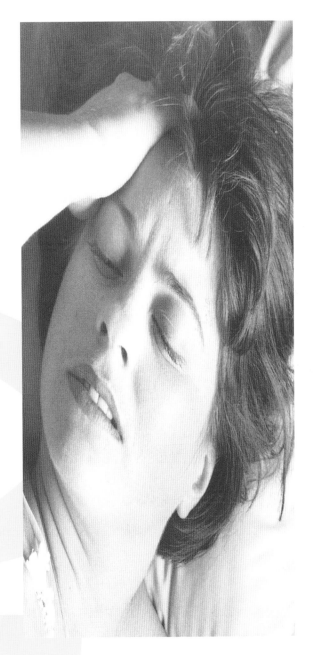

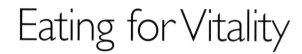

Eating for Vitality

Food is the fuel that drives your body. Without enough of the right nutrients you will lose strength and vitality.

The three basic nutrients obtained through foods are carbohydrates, fats, and proteins. Fiber, vitamins, minerals, as well as trace elements, enzymes, and so on, are also extracted by our bodies from the food we eat and are essential to our well-being.

Many people believe protein is the main source of energy in the diet. The truth is, however, that carbohydrates, and to a lesser extent fats, supply the body with energy, to keep the organs — including the nervous system — working and muscles active, and for any activity we undertake. Protein is essential to the growth and maintenance of the body. We need 25–30 grams of protein daily to sustain good health. Animal sources of protein are meat products, poultry, fish, milk, and eggs.

Soybeans have a higher protein content than lean meat, and peanuts, almonds, buckwheat, sunflower seeds, pumpkin seeds, potatoes, avocados, and sprouted legumes (peas, beans and lentils) are all rich protein sources. Plant proteins are more easily digested than animal proteins, and are rich sources of complex carbohydrates — starches and sugars — and other nutrients such as vitamins, minerals, fat, and the fiber necessary for the elimination of waste products, including toxins. These complex carbohydrate foods are slow to break down to their final component of simple sugars, so they release a constant stream of glucose into the bloodstream over a period of time — this ensures lasting high energy levels.

Good quality fats from vegetable sources should not be scorned by anyone, even those wanting to lose weight. They are converted into fatty acids during digestion and are vital for making membranes and hormones and for proper functioning of the brain; they are as well an easily assimilable form of food energy.

14

High Energy Whole Foods

Grains, seeds, and nuts contain all the important nutrients essential for growth and maintaining good health, including essential fatty acids that are necessary for reducing fatigue and increasing energy levels.

Seeds are the highest protein vegetable food and contain nearly all 10 essential amino acids. The protein content of seeds is richer than meat. They should be eaten raw, but need to be thoroughly chewed before swallowing. Other methods of breaking seeds down are soaking overnight, grinding in a coffee mill to sprinkle over breakfast cereals, or liquefying in a blender as part of a health drink.

Note: Sunflower seeds should be gray in color; yellow, brown, white, or black seeds are rancid and therefore toxic.

Nuts must be eaten fresh and raw. The most nutritious are almonds, peanuts, and hazelnuts.

Grains which are best for increasing energy levels are buckwheat and millet. The proteins in buckwheat are comparable to the proteins in meat. It is necessary to cook grains to release all the vital minerals. Sprouting grains also releases the minerals.

Beans or legumes should not be eaten raw. Soybeans are the highest source of complete protein.

Avocados contain complete nutrition — protein, fats, carbohydrates, minerals, and vitamins.

Mushrooms are low in calories and a good source of vitamins, particularly the B group, and are high in riboflavin, niacin and pantothenic acid. They are a good source of minerals, especially potassium and copper. Because of their essential amino acid content, 70–90% of mushroom protein can be easily digested. Eat them raw or lightly cooked.

Potatoes are high in protein as well as in complex carbohydrates.

Sprouts

Seeds, grains, and beans contain the living germ of the plant, so are "live foods." When sprouted, their vitamin and mineral content is significantly increased. Alfalfa, mung beans, sunflower seeds, lentils, buckwheat, millet, and rye are ideal for sprouting.

Note: In the entries on herbs, food supplements, vitamins and minerals in the following pages, only those properties relating to the body's energy levels are listed.

Herbs for Promoting Energy

Alfalfa is one of the most complete foods available. It contains important enzymes, proteins, minerals, and vitamins. Alfalfa helps counteract fatigue, toxins, and acidity.

Dandelion makes a healthy tonic for the liver and gallbladder. It is a digestive aid and a powerful blood cleanser and tonic.

Echinacea is a blood purifying herb, and has a tonic effect on the lymphatic system and glands. Echinacea is especially useful for restoring vitality in people recovering from illness.

Fo-ti-tieng assists better absorption of foods in the digestive system and increases metabolism. It improves energy, memory, resistance to mental fatigue, and is a brain food.

Garlic contains special sugar-regulating factors, 17 amino acids, 33 sulphur compounds, vitamins A, C, and B1, plus trace amounts of selenium and germanium. To eliminate the odor on your breath, eat a fresh and large sized sprig of parsley, stalks and all — it does work!

Ginseng is a general tonic and blood purifier. It can be used in the treatment of anemia and other blood diseases, depression, and blood sugar problems. It promotes mental and physical vitality, relief of stress and insomnia, and good digestion. It is especially useful following an illness.

Licorice is a good liver-cleansing herb.

Milk thistle is effective for lack of appetite and dyspepsia, as well as being good for the liver, gallbladder, and spleen.

Parsley is an excellent source of iron and vitamin C. It is effective in the treatment of anemia and its symptoms, fatigue, irritability, and general debility. It is also a valuable liver cleanser and is an effective digestant.

The Energy Tricksters — Coffee, Tea, Sugar and Alcohol

All the above give us a high, an immediate burst of energy, a feeling we can cope with just about anything. When we're feeling down, one of the first things that enters our minds is "I need a coffee/tea/drink/some chocolate…"

However, the effect of this instant energy wears off quickly and you may be left feeling lower in energy, less able to cope, than you did before. Coffee and tea stimulate the adrenal glands. This causes the liver to release a burst of sugar into the bloodstream. Sugar pumps glucose straight into the bloodstream, dangerously raising blood sugar levels. An excess of insulin is then shot into the bloodstream, causing a sudden lowering of blood sugar to levels below normal. The pancreas, the liver, and the adrenal glands are now under stress. Energy levels are substantially lowered and your emotional stability is affected. Alcohol is a concentrated form of carbohydrate and produces the same effect as sugar. Also, it drains the body of magnesium, a mineral essential for energy.

Dried fruits — figs, apricots, papaya, raisins, sultanas — and carob are nutritious substitutes for candy. They should be introduced gradually to wean you or your child from harmful sweets. Once you have become used to these flavors, you will find regular confectionaries unpalatable.

Care For Your Liver

The liver is the body's major detoxifying organ and the main organ of food metabolism. Among its many functions, the liver stores and regulates the amount of blood sugar the body draws on for energy. A glass of pure water with the juice of half a lemon morning and night, and plenty of pure water during the day will help keep your liver in good working order.

There is no substitute for a well-balanced diet of fresh foods.

Preparing Your Own Fast Foods

Busy people often eat commercially prepared food or fast foods because they feel they don't have time to cook each night. The answer is to create your own "fast foods." Once a month or every two weeks — depending on your or your family's needs — cook large pots of soups, stew, or pasta sauces, or bake several pies, to be divided into many meal-sized portions. These can then be put into the freezer and taken out as needed. For variety, keep a few different dishes always ready for the microwave, oven or hotplate. Add a tossed salad (always use cold-pressed oils for salad dressings) and your healthy meal is prepared with no more effort than putting a pre-packaged meal into the microwave.

For salad dressings, always use unrefined, cold-pressed oils from your health food store. Sesame seed oil and olive oil are perhaps the best choices, as they are slow to go rancid and contain many health-giving nutrients. Store in your refrigerator.

Some Recipes for Energy

Banana Power Whip

1 large banana
2 teaspoons sunflower seeds or almond nuts
1/4 teaspoon brewer's yeast (gradually increase to 1 teaspoon)
1 teaspoon dolomite powder
1/4 cup wheatgerm
1/4 cup bran (wheat, oat, barley)
enough milk (soy, skim, or low fat) to right consistency for you.

Put all ingredients into a blender and put on high speed until frothy. Pour into a large glass and drink. For variety, add some chopped apple or pear, or strawberries into the mixture. This makes an excellent breakfast.

Lentil Stew

14 1/2 oz (450 g) lentils
5 slices well-trimmed bacon
2 stalks celery (chopped)
2 young carrots (chopped)
1 medium capsicum red
   or green (diced)
2 medium potatoes
2 medium onions (chopped)
3–5 cloves garlic (chopped)
1 teaspoon sea salt
2 teaspoons cold-pressed olive oil

Sauté onions in olive oil until clear. Add all other ingredients, except the garlic, into a large pot, and cover with cold water. Put on high heat until boiling, then reduce heat. Simmer for 1 hour then add garlic. Add more sea salt if required. Simmer for a further 1/2 hour if necessary. Divide into 8 portions, put into plastic containers, and place in the freezer until required.

Green Rice

1 lb (500 g) of parsley
1 lb (500 g) of brown rice
1 lb (500 g) of fat-reduced
shredded cheddar cheese
2 medium onions
3–5 cloves garlic
Juice of 1 lemon
1/2 teaspoon sea salt (if required)

While boiling brown rice for 30 minutes, pinch off parsley leaves and discard the stalks. Wash parsley leaves in cold water and drain. In your food processor, finely chop garlic and onions and put into a large bowl. Chop parsley leaves in the food processor and add to the garlic and onions. Add salt to the lemon juice, then pour into the bowl. Mix all ingredients well. Add shredded cheese and mix well with other ingredients. Once the rice has boiled for 30 minutes, drain. Put the rice back into the pot and add other ingredients. Mix well, until all the rice turns green. Spoon into 5 personal casserole dishes (large helpings) or 7 (smaller helpings).

If you only have 1 or 2 personal casserole dishes, the other helpings can be put into plastic containers. Put into the freezer. To defrost, take a serving from the freezer in the morning before going to work, or defrost using your microwave. Bake in the oven set at 400° F (200° C) for 30 minutes or until brown on top.

Diet Supplements for Fatigue

The following concentrated food supplements can be purchased in tablet, capsule, liquid, or powder form from your health food store.

Concentrated Food Supplement	How It Affects Your Energy Levels	Nutrients
Blackstrap molasses	Excellent tonic for the blood, helps build red blood cells which carry oxygen around the body.	Excellent source of many essential minerals (esp. iron & potassium) as well as vitamin E and the B-complex vitamins.
Brewer's yeast	Assists the body in retaining health and energy. Special benefit to those who suffer extreme nervous or physical strain. Take ¼ tsp to begin gradually increasing to tablespoon per day. Should be taken with dolomite (calcium).	Vitamins B1, B2, B3, B5, B6, calcium, iron, potassium, protein, carbohydrate, amino acids, small amount of fat. Caution: do not confuse with active Baker's yeast.
Chlorophyll	Green substance in plants which transforms the sun's energy into food sugars. Helps build red blood cells and is a useful liver tonic. Taken as directed, it significantly increases energy levels.	Rich in enzymes, vitamins, minerals, and trace minerals, its chemical components are almost the same as those in human blood. Best natural sources are alfalfa, barley and wheat grass.
Desiccated liver	Increases stamina and energy, and is an effective anti-stress food. Tonic for general good health.	Simply dried beef liver, this is one of the best sources of B vitamins, vitamin A and trace minerals.
Dolomite	Strengthens bones and teeth. Necessary for weight-bearing exercise and general good health. It also calms the nerves.	Naturally occurring source of calcium and magnesium found in crystals or rock, microrefined and sterilized.

Fiber	Assists in the elimination of waste products, including toxins. A sluggish system will make you tired and listless. Guar gum stabilizes blood sugar levels.	Wheat, rice, oat, barley brans, guar gum, linseed, and psyllium husks are good fiber supplements.
Ginkgo biloba	Species of tree that has survived over 200 million years. It is used as an antioxidant, and increases alertness and general feeling of well-being. Helps depression and improves energy levels.	Flavoglycosides are the active ingredients and promote better circulation.
Kelp	Assists the thyroid gland produce the hormone thyroxine. Its tonic effect helps reduce fatigue and lethargy.	Rich in vitamins, minerals (esp. iodine), and trace elements.
Lecithin	Balances and distributes fats throughout the body. Useful in the treatment of diseases of the liver, circulatory system, and blood disorders. A deficiency can cause fatigue, insomnia, and nervous tension.	Soybeans, egg yolk, corn.
Spirulina	A powerhouse of nutrients in the form of microscopic blue-green algae that substantially and quickly increases energy and stamina, among its many contributions to human health.	Essential source of vitamin B12, rich source of iron, protein, calcium, GLA, vitamin E, chromium, chlorophyll, beta-carotene, phosphorus, potassium, calcium, magnesium, and zinc.
Wheat germ	A whole food whose reproductive power is vital for general health and well-being.	Rich in protein, oils, B-vitamins, vitamin E, iron, magnesium, zinc, and other nutrients. Beware of rancid wheat germ.

Vitamins, Minerals, and Trace Elements

It is important to note that neither vitamins nor minerals provide energy. They do, however, aid the transfer of energy from carbohydrate, fat, and protein to body organs. Vitamins are much more effective if consumed in their natural form in food or in supplement tablets derived from natural food sources, e.g. beta-carotene or cod liver oil capsules for vitamin A, brewer's yeast tablets or powder for B-complex, dolomite powder or tablets for calcium. Minerals should be purchased in their chelated forms to ensure effective absorption.

Supplement	How it Affects Your Energy Levels	Some Better Food Sources
Vitamins	*Essential to normal metabolism*	*All natural foods*
B-complex — B1 thiamine, B2 riboflavin, B3 niacin, B5 pantothenic acid, B6 pyridoxine, biotin, folic acid, and B12 cyanocobalamin	Maintains the nervous system. Essential for assimilation of carbohydrates and protein. Assists the liver and adrenal glands, therefore sugar metabolism. Good for bad nerves, stress, muscular weakness, mental fatigue, and vitality. B5 & B6 are especially important to people with low blood sugar.	Brewer's yeast, grains, nuts, and seeds (esp. sesame, pumpkin, and flax), mushrooms, blackstrap molasses.
Vitamin C	Essential for iron absorption and the maintenance of healthy red blood cells. Builds resistance to illness. An antioxidant, it helps protect against stress and toxins. Best taken with bioflavonoids.	Guavas, capsicums, blackcurrants, parsley, Brussels sprouts, broccoli, watercress, cantaloupe, red cabbage, other fruits and vegetables.
Co-Enzyme Q10	Also known as Vitamin Q. Manufactures ATP which is the basic energy molecule of cells. Called the "cellular spark plug" it is extremely effective in boosting, then maintaining, energy levels and improving circulation.	Available in small amounts in food supply, but beef heart is a particularly rich source.
Vitamin E	Improves oxygen supply to cells. Protects pituitary and adrenal hormones and adrenal cortex.	Wheat germ, rice germ, whole grains, cold-pressed oils, seeds, nuts, and beans, green leafy vegetables, salmon, lamb's liver.

Minerals and Trace Elements	Deficiency can lead to lack of energy and general ill health.	All natural foods
Calcium	Strengthens bones and teeth. Necessary for weight-bearing exercise and general good health.	Dolomite, cheese, dietary yeast, carob powder, soy milk, parsley, nuts, sardines, dairy products, blackstrap molasses.
Chromium	Assists in the conversion of sugar and transfer of glucose from the blood into the body.	Brewer's and nutritional yeast.
Iodine	Essential for health of thyroid gland and the hormone thyroxine. Lack will cause anemia, fatigue, low blood pressure, lethargy, and thyroid problems.	Kelp, cranberries.
Iron	Involved in the formation of red blood cells. Maintains oxygen stores within red blood cells, and assists the memory and ability to concentrate. Aids resistance to stress and fatigue. Essential in the chemical reactions that produce energy from food. Take with vitamin C to ensure absorption.	Beef, liver, haddock, cod, spirulina, dietary yeasts, rice bran, wheat bran, wheatgerm, beans, seeds, nuts, eggs, parsley, blackstrap molasses.
Magnesium	Necessary for normal muscular activity. Works with calcium in metabolism. It performs an important role in energy release and the functioning of nerves.	Nuts and grains (esp. buckwheat), soybeans, dolomite, dried fruits, molasses, fresh fruits and vegetables.
Manganese	Assists in the formation of thyroid hormone, thyroxine, and the manufacture of insulin. Involved in the metabolism of carbohydrates and proteins, and utilization of fats.	Grains (esp. buckwheat), alfalfa sprouts, nuts, avocado, parsley, carrots, green vegetables, beetroot, egg yolk.
Potassium	Good for extreme fatigue, muscular weakness, irritability, depression.	Blackstrap molasses, grains, brewer's yeast, soybeans, bananas, dried fruits, sunflower seeds, cranberries.
Zinc	Regulates insulin activity. A deficiency may cause lethargy, apathy, loss of appetite.	Liver, lean meat, poultry, buckwheat, nuts, seeds, cheese, fish, meat.
Trace Minerals	Can be toxic if taken in too large amounts. Best to use a chelated multi-mineral complex.	Parsley, kelp, alfalfa, dolomite, nutritional yeast, watercress.

Get Your Body Moving

Exercise is vital to good health and vitality. It helps keep bones and muscles strong, improves circulation, increases the amount of oxygen in the blood, reduces stress, makes you less prone to anxiety and depression, and improves your alertness and vitality.

You do not have to do huge amounts of exercise every day — even the so-called required 30 minutes three times a week can be off-putting to a busy person. Exercise should be, above all things, fun. If you see it as a chore, you are either very busy or very tired, or you haven't found the right exercise for you. If the former is the case, then you need to review your diet and workload for starters. There are many different activities you can do, at home, out in the open air, or at a club. Whatever form of exercise you choose, begin in a small way. Over time you'll find that you gradually build the time and effort you put into it, not because you should, but because you want to — exercise does become addictive.

Walking is a pleasant, no-stress exercise that is extremely effective. Jogging is exhilarating, but does require some fitness. Swimming exercises every muscle in the body, while cycling and dancing are both good cardiovascular activities than can be done either alone or with friends.

Whatever exercise you choose to do, it is important to start moving. Do a few minutes of stretching when you get out of bed in the morning, then make a choice to walk an extra block before catching the bus, even if it means getting up half an hour earlier. Perhaps you could use the stairs instead of the elevator. Whatever you decide, try to make the activity a regular, day-to-day routine.

A Routine for the Office

You can exercise while sitting in your chair in the office. Most people are constantly bent over keyboards or writing pads — and this is very bad for your back, neck, and shoulders.

For your neck

Sit up straight in your chair, then flop your head forward. Intertwine your fingers behind your head, just above your neck, your elbows forward, and pull down gently. Hold for a few seconds, then lift your head up again, and let it flop backwards, the back of your chair taking the weight of your body. While your head is in this position, shake it gently, then raise your head upright. Sit, keeping your shoulders back and down. Next, turn your head to the right. With one hand on your chin, the other behind your head, turn your head as far as it can go. Repeat with other side. Do these neck stretches every so often during the day or when you are feeling strain in your neck.

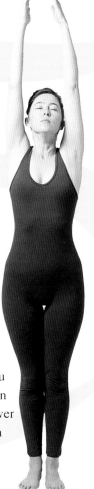

No Pain, No Gain?

Exercise should not cause you pain. Pain is a warning that something is wrong and you should stop that activity immediately. Warming up before the exercise and cooling down afterward helps prevent muscular pain or injury. Stretching or shaking out your muscles after each sequence of movements will help keep your muscles relaxed.

For your back and shoulders

While sitting in your chair, stretch both arms up toward the ceiling as far as you can. Hold, push back slightly, return to center, then lower your arms to the desk. Sit, keeping your shoulders back and down. Now stand. Lift yourself onto your toes and stretch to the ceiling as far as you can go. Hold for several seconds, then relax, and lower your arms as you lower your feet to the floor. Shake out each leg, then shake your arms as though they were limp ropes.

Some Basic Stretching Exercises

Stretching loosens muscles and joints, and improves flexibility. It is an essential start to any exercise routine to prevent injury, as well as being an energy booster at the beginning of the day.

1. Stand with feet shoulder-width apart, knees slightly bent, back straight, arms hanging loosely by your sides. Take a few deep breaths.

2. Straighten your body and tense your legs. As you inhale, raise your arms in an arc from your sides to reach for the ceiling. As you do this, raise yourself onto your toes. Reach up toward the ceiling, stretching your toes, your legs, your torso, your arms, your fingers. Hold for a few moments.

4. As you exhale, slowly lower your arms to your side; at the same time, lower your heels to the floor, and allow your body to relax.

5. Shake tension out of each leg and each arm. Repeat exercise three times.

6. Stand with feet about three feet (1 m) apart. As you inhale, raise your right arm above your head. At the same time, reach your left arm down your leg as far as you can without straining.

7. Exhale, and return to upright position. Shake out each leg and each arm. Repeat steps 6 and 7 with the other arm. Repeat exercise three times.

8. Stand with your feet about three feet (1 m) apart, your knees bent. Inhale and raise your arms out to the side until they are level with your shoulders. Exhale.

9. The following movement should be conducted as one smooth action. Inhale, and in a slow, sweeping action, swing your upper torso around to the right, bending your knees slightly and exhaling as you do. Your upper torso is now twisted around so you are facing behind you, legs straight. Hold for a moment. Inhale and, as you slowly swing your upper torso back to center, continue the swing to the other side, again bending your knees and exhaling. Your upper torso is now twisted around so you are facing behind you. Hold for a moment. As you swing back to center, inhale, straighten your knees and hold your arms out to the side, level with your shoulders.

10. As you exhale, lower your arms to your sides. Repeat exercise three times.

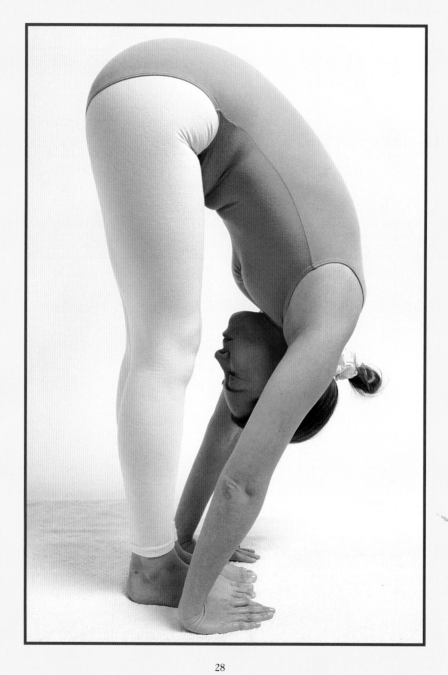

A Quick Morning Session

From the standing position

1. Bounce from your toes up and down on the spot 50 times. Let your arms flap and jiggle as they will. Be aware of your shoulders, let them move freely. Glide your attention over the rest of your body, moving down the arms, over the abdomen. Any place that is stiff, let flop. Allow your body to behave like jelly. Visualize all your bones and muscles and body organs as separate entities bouncing within the confines of your body.

2. Jog on the spot 50 times (count left leg only) to begin with, gradually increasing the number as your fitness improves. Don't attempt to raise your knees high at this stage, but as your leg muscles get stronger, you can raise your knees higher.

3. Stand upright. Lift your left knee and clasp your hands around it. Pull it close to your chest. Hold for a moment, then release. Stand upright. Lift your right knee and clasp your hands around it. Pull it close to your chest. Hold for a moment, then release. Repeat three times.

4. Stand upright, your knees bent, your feet shoulder-width apart. Loosen your shoulders. Move your left foot forward, then swing your right arm in full circles, 10 times to begin with. Then swing back the other way, 10 times. Shake out shoulders. Move your right foot forward and repeat exercise with your left arm. Gradually increase the number of circles to 20 forward and 20 backward. This exercise is particularly good for keeping neck and shoulder muscles flexible.

5. Stand upright, feet shoulder-width apart. Inhale, then exhale and bend from the hips, rolling your torso down over your knees, until you feel your back and hamstring muscles begin to stretch. Hold for 10 to 20 seconds, breathing normally. But do not try to touch your toes at first. You will quickly become flexible enough to be able to do so without strain. Inhale and raise yourself upright. Shake out each leg and each arm. Repeat 10 times.

6. Do 20 star jumps. Then shake out each leg and each arm.

On the floor

1. Lie on your left side and, inhaling, raise right leg as high as you can without strain. Hold for a few seconds, then exhale and lower your leg to the floor. Repeat 5 times. Lie on your right side and, inhaling, raise your left leg as high as you can without strain. Hold for a few seconds, then exhale and lower your leg to the floor. Repeat 5 times.

2. Lie on your stomach, your hands on the floor near your shoulders. Inhale and push yourself up by your hands and knees. Make sure your back is straight. As you exhale, slowly lower your chest to the ground by bending your arms at the elbows. Inhale, and raise yourself onto your hands and knees. Repeat 5 times.

3. On your hands and knees, your back straight, raise your right leg up so that your thigh is parallel to your torso, your lower leg pointing upward. Hold for a few seconds, then slowly lower to the ground. Raise your left leg up so that your thigh is parallel to your torso. Hold for a few seconds, then slowly lower to the round. Repeat exercise 5 times.

Step 1

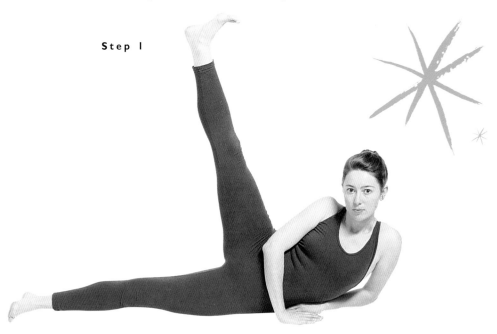

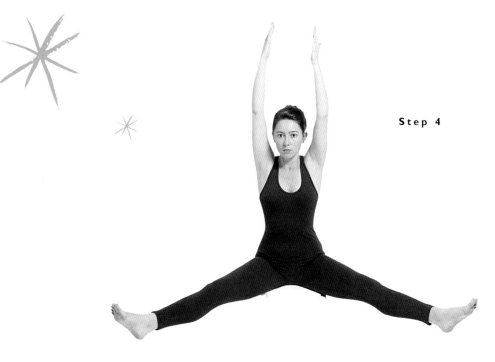

4. Sitting on the floor, spread your legs as wide as you can in front of you. As you inhale, raise both arms above your head.

5. As you exhale, lower your body over your right leg and grasp your leg as close to the ankle as possible. Hold for a few seconds. Inhale and bring your body back to upright position. Exhale. Inhale and raise both arms above your head. As you exhale, lower your body over your left leg and grasp your leg as close to the ankle as possible. Hold for a few seconds. Inhale and bring your body back to upright position. Repeat exercise 5 times.

Step 5

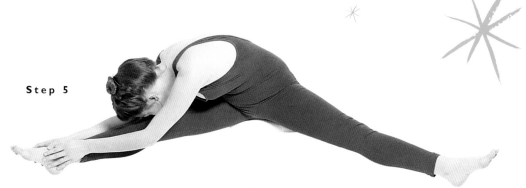

You Are What You Think

We think, then we act. Everything we do, everything we say,
is the result of our thinking.

People who hold the attitude "If I don't expect much, then I won't be disappointed" generally have rather dull lives and lack get up and go. The reason for this is that what you expect in life is usually what you get.

Enthusiasm instantly creates energy, just as surely as disappointment destroys it. You have control over the way you think; therefore you have control over the quality of your day-to-day life.

A Tendency to Overreact

Do you have a tendency to suffer setbacks on a regular basis? Does life seem to treat you harshly?

To find the answer, pick a recent day that was particularly upsetting to you and write down everything that caused you distress. Pretend these things happened to a friend of yours and she or he is telling you about them. Your friend's tone is distressed, perhaps a little whiny. Notice how your friend is breathing — short, sharp breaths. See how the hands are moving around, clenching and unclenching. See the tension in the body.

As you observe, what are your thoughts about your friend's reaction to these events? Do these events justify the amount of distress and energy being expended here? The time has come to advise your friend. What are you going to say?

> *Visualize a project completed.*
> *Imagine yourself doing it.*
> *Do it!*

"Lighten Up" — Becoming Optimistic

"Lighten up" is a colloquial expression that means exactly what it says. Negative thinking is a heavy burden. It literally bends the body and drains the energy every bit as much as would carrying a heavy weight.

Have you ever said: "I can't achieve that, why should I even bother?" It would have been preferable to say: "How do I know I can't do that, if I don't even try?" Here is the beginning of optimism, but there is still an element of doubt. Inherent in this statement is the notion that though I am willing to give it a go, I reserve to right to give up if I find the going difficult. An even better thought would be: "I know that if I can visualize it, I can make it happen. I know this because if I didn't have the ability to make it happen, I wouldn't be able to see it — the brain and the body only do what the mind tells them to do. All I need now is to find out *how* to achieve my goal."

Can You Say "No"?

If we take on too much at the same time, we will become tired and irritable, we could even burn out. Many people have difficulty saying "no" when asked to do something, and before they know it, they're up till all hours baking for the school fete as well as making costumes for the school play, or they've taken home work yet again to cover for their lazy colleague. When someone asks you to take on something or before you are tempted to offer your services, ask yourself what are your current commitments and plans for relaxation and do you really have the time to take on this extra burden. If not, say: "I'm sorry, I'm really caught up right now." You will be amazed at how easily people accept this without argument or bad feeling.

When You Find Yourself Thinking Negatively...

- Is there a positive option? Visualize yourself in that space.
- When a negative image enters your mind, replace it with a joyful one.
- Recall some event that gave you pleasure and relive it.
- Don't let the behavior of others get you down.
- Forget about what you can't change.
- Be kind to yourself — remember, no one is perfect.
- Feel the wonder and power in each present moment.
- Be glad to be alive and vibrant and ready for anything.

Positive Self-Talk

I can see myself achieving my goal. I can see myself working on [the project], and it is difficult. But that makes it a challenge and I find the notion of challenge exciting. No one ever achieved anything worthwhile who didn't undertake a challenge. No one created a great work of art, made a lot of money, climbed the corporate ladder, was a good parent or a loving, supportive spouse without effort, sacrifice, and the desire to surmount obstacles. No one came out of the womb with all their skills and knowledge intact — these had to be earned and strived for.

I know I will make mistakes — everyone makes mistakes when they're trying to achieve something — but I will be able to learn from them and move forward. While making mistakes is frustrating — sometimes even making me feel stupid — solving even the tiniest element of a problem is exhilarating and makes me feel I've achieved something wonderful. And while I am enjoying solving all these problems, I'm getting ever closer to seeing my [project] complete.

Dealing with Difficulties

Trouble comes to all people no matter who they are or what they've got. When a positive thinker, an optimistic person, comes up against adversity, they try to remain cheerful and refuse to believe this adversity can undo them. They recognize the problem for what it is, and know that where there is a problem, there is a solution. When a negative thinker comes up against adversity, they believe their world is crashing down and there is nothing to be done. They are crushed by the weight of their own negativity.

Try not to let trouble overwhelm you. At first, the shock of the situation will disorient you. At this time it is best to keep still. This is a good time to practice the arts of aromatherapy, breathing, yoga, and massage. Some gentle, non-demanding meditation will also help restore your clarity and composure.

Ask questions about your problem to establish just how serious it is and what elements are involved. Once you have grasped the situation, your choices will become clearer and you will know the best action to take.

Accept losses or situations that can't be changed, and let them go. It is no use worrying about something over which you have no control.

Be Kind to Yourself

Release Some Tension

Throw a tantrum! Pound the floor rapidly. Jump up and down while clenching your fists and moaning, groaning, yelling, screaming. Put everything you have into it and don't stop until you are spent.

How do you feel? Absolutely fabulous? If not, do it again.

Pounding a pillow, hitting a punching bag, screaming in the car, or shouting in the shower, will have similar effects. With the heavy weight of tension lifted, your body should feel light and full of energy, ready to undertake even the most onerous task!

Don't panic. Where there is a problem, there is always a solution.

We all have faults. If we were perfect, we would be in heaven, not here. Beating yourself up over your faults will do no one any good, least of all you. The best way to overcome your negative impulses is to be relaxed and cheerful, not dwelling on your faults — your sincere desire to overcome them is enough. This in turn will create positive, cheerful actions, and the faults, deprived of nourishment from your thoughts, will whither and die, leaving you happy and energized.

The Importance of Breath

Breathing is the most important function of your body. Without oxygen you would die in minutes. Oxygen is essential for the life of every organ and cell in your body. It is essential for energy. The more efficiently oxygen can get to body cells, the more alert you will be.

Our sedentary lifestyles greatly affect how much oxygen we take in and how well it is absorbed. Apart from getting sufficient exercise, we also need to learn how to breathe properly. Eastern mystical disciplines, like meditation, yoga, and t'ai chi, place the most important emphasis on breath and its control. With each breath, we take in essential energy or life force (known by the Hindus as prana, by the Chinese as chi) and with each exhalation, stagnant energies are expelled.

A Yogic Breathing Exercise

Correct breathing will be difficult for you if, like most people, you breathe in a shallow manner. Breathing deeply and fully can make you dizzy if you are not used to it, so it may be best to begin by lying flat on the floor, or on a bed with a firm mattress, with your arms by your sides, your palms facing upward. Breathe in through the nose and exhale from your mouth. Until you are comfortable with the technique, place your hand over the part of the lung area to which you are directing the air — this way, you will be able to tell whether the air is reaching that part. Close your eyes.

1. Place your hands over your abdomen. As you slowly breathe in to the count of 8, mentally direct the flow of air to the bottom of your lungs beneath your rib cage. You may not be able to reach that far at first, so take the breath as far as you can. Your abdomen should expand as the air reaches the lower parts of your lungs. Hold the breath for a count of 8, then exhale slowly to the count of 8, vocalizing "ahhhhhh" until there is no more air to expel.

2. Place your hands on your rib cage. As you breathe in to a count of 8, mentally direct the air so that it pushes your rib cage outward. Hold the breath for a count of 8, then exhale slowly to the count of 8, vocalizing "ahhhhhh" until there is no more air to expel.

3. Place your hands on your shoulders. As you breathe in to a count of 8, mentally direct the air to your upper lungs. You should feel your shoulders expand. Hold the breath for a count of 8, then exhale slowly to the count of 8, vocalizing "ahhhhhh" until there is no more air to expel.

Once you are comfortable with the three stages described above, try incorporating all three stages into one long breath.

4. Breathe in to the count of 9, filling the abdomen first (1,2,3), then the rib cage (4,5,6), and finally the shoulder region (7,8,9). Hold the breath for the count of 9. Exhale from the shoulder region (1,2,3), from the rib cage (4,5,6) from the abdomen (7,8,9).

    The next step is to practice this controlled breathing technique while sitting on the floor, cross-legged, in the lotus position, or half-lotus position, in preparation for meditation or deep relaxation.

Note: Do not be dismayed if you can't reach the count of 8 or 9 — it will take practice. Start with a count of say 5. The important thing is that your breathing is controlled. Take the same count for breathing in, holding the breath, and for breathing out.

Alternate Nostril Breath

This is a very tranquil practice. It rids the body of toxins, balances the flow of energy and expels stale air. The brain cells are enlivened. It is important to keep the inhalation and exhalation the same length. Try counting: one, two, three, one, two, three ...You may notice one nostril is more blocked than the other. This is usually the case. The practice of Nadi Shodhan ensures each nostril gets a turn — this is very important as breathing predominantly through one side can lead to disharmony in the body.

1. Using your right hand, place index and middle fingers on your brow, centered between your eyes. Let your thumb rest beside your right nostril, and your ring finger beside your left nostril.

2. Block the right nostril with your thumb and inhale through the left nostril. Draw the breath up toward the center of your eyebrows. Make the breath slow and even.

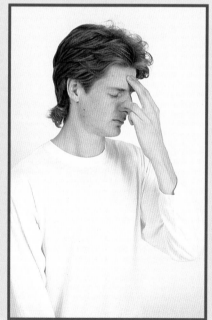

3. Now, block off the left nostril with your ring finger and exhale through the right.

4. Once all the air is expelled, inhale through the right nostril, keeping the left nostril blocked.

5. This time exhale through the left nostril, blocking the right.

6. Continue the practice, breathing in through one nostril and out the other. As you practice, see if you can lengthen the time of each breath in and out. However, never let yourself become out of breath. If you experience any discomfort, cease the practice and rest.

Humming Bee Breath

The Humming Bee Breath is an exhilarating way to clear the mind of excess clutter. Our ability to think clearly is frequently undermined by random thoughts racing around the mind. This exercise quells negative emotions such as anger and anxiety, and helps lower blood pressure. The Humming Bee Breath also strengthens the voice box.

1. Inhale, and place your index fingers in your ears, thus blocking out the noises of the world.

2. As you exhale, make a humming, buzzing sound with your mouth. Keep your mouth closed. Pretend you are a bee. Feel the sound reverberate in the front of your brain. Extend the exhalation as long as you can. Keep your fingers in your ears as you exhale.

3. Repeat the breath several times.

Awareness

Experience the vibration of the sound throughout your mind. Be aware of nothing else.
When you finish the practice, notice how your mind is crisp and lucid. Whenever you feel "frazzled," try the Humming Bee Breath.

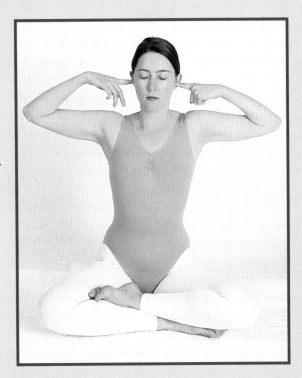

Deep Relaxation for Energy

Deep relaxation means to deeply relax the mind and body.
It helps to center your being, creating harmony and balance.
To boost your energy levels over the long term, it is vital to
incorporate some form of regular deep relaxation into your life.

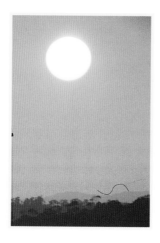

The exercise below is a simple one. Practiced before retiring at night, it will improve your sleep; practiced first thing in the morning, it will increase your energy levels. Spend 15 minutes morning and night if you can, but even 5 minutes each morning and night will transform your sense of self, your mental clarity, and your ability to control your reactions to life's events.

If the idea of total silence does not appeal to you, you can play soft music in the background to help you relax and focus. The music can be chosen from the MUSIC FOR FOCUSING selection on page 75, or you can buy tapes and CDs especially designed for the purpose of meditation and relaxation — these often include sounds from nature. A candle scented with essential oils also helps create a harmonious atmosphere. You may like to put this exercise on tape, to guide you through your relaxation.

Lie on the floor and close your eyes. Become aware of yourself... your body... on the floor... in the room... Allow yourself to become aware of any noises around you... in the room... outside the room... Don't try to stop any sounds, just allow them to flow in... and out... Become aware of your breathing... Focus on your lungs as you breathe in... and feel them expand... As you breathe out, feel your lungs contract... breathe in... breathe out... Be aware as you focus on your breathing how it becomes slower... and deeper... Now spend a little time focusing on your breathing... Don't try to force your breath, just become aware of it as you breathe in... and out...

As you breathe in, imagine your breath as a light-filled vapor, expanding from your lungs... until it fills your body... breathe out... as you breathe in become aware of any tensions in your body... breathe out... breathe in and direct your breath to a point of tension and imagine your breath, as light-filled vapor, absorbing that tension... breathe out, knowing your breath is taking the tension with it, out of your body...

And now become aware of your breath... As you breathe in... and out... in... and out... become aware of your body on the floor... in the room... As your breathing normalizes, become aware of the noises within the room... outside the room... become aware of your body in the room... and become aware of the feeling in your body... in your fingers... your toes... And as you come back to the room... to the present time... and place... be aware that — at any time — whenever it is needed, whenever you need to become calm, relaxed, and peaceful, your breath can absorb and expel your tensions.

When you are fully present, open your eyes and sit up.

The Vital Energy of Yoga

The purpose of yoga is to unify the physical body with the mind and with the vital energy flowing within it, thus you can experience a sense of harmony and balance.

Yoga encourages a strong body, a sharp mind, and it reduces stress. If you practice yoga on a daily basis, along with yogic breathing exercises and meditation, you will find that problems you once considered overwhelming to be little more than a hiccup in the course of an otherwise fruitful and fulfilling life. The following set of positions calms tensions and increases energy.

Arm and Shoulder Lift

This yoga posture gently stretches the shoulders and arms, while the body rests. It increases energy levels and activates the immune system.

1. Sit on your heels, your knees close together — if you can't sit on your heels, put a cushion between you and your legs and sit on it instead. Rest the toes of one foot on the other, so that the toes are touching, but the heels are apart. Rest your hands in your lap. Lengthen your spine and hold your head upright. This is known as the Thunderbolt pose.

2. Lower your head until it touches the floor in front of your knees. Clasp your hands together behind your back.

3. As you inhale, begin to lift your arms, hands clasped, away from your back. With your arms in a straight line, move them toward your head, pointing toward the ceiling, as far as possible without strain. Exhale, and breathe normally in the position for a few moments.

4. Inhale and move your arms a little further toward your head.

5. Exhale and lower your arms to rest on the floor. You are now resting in the Pose of the Child.

Work gradually with this posture. You should never jerk your arms or force them in any way, but move only as you feel the muscles release.

Regular yoga practice not only strengthens your body; it strengthens your mind, your emotions, and your spirit.

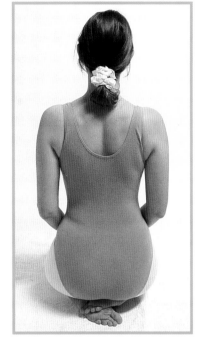

Step 1

Step 3

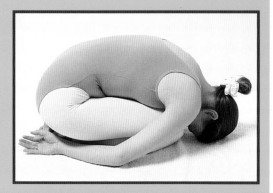

Pose of the child

The Pose of the Child

The Pose of the Child is a resting position that is particularly soothing for tight back muscles. This pose is very restorative if you are experiencing anxiety or feeling depleted. It calms the mind and emotions, and restores energy. It also regulates adrenal gland function and tones the pelvic region and sexual organs.

A variation: Stretch your arms out in front of you, palms facing downwards. This will extend the back muscles.

Variation on Pose of the Child

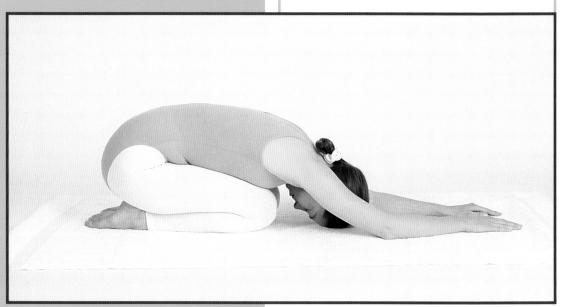

The Cat

The Cat stretch is one of the most relaxing of all the yoga poses. It loosens and stretches the entire spinal column. It is, as well, an excellent posture if you have been sitting at a desk all day. Pay special attention to your breathing during this exercise. Always breathe in deeply as you arch your back, and exhale fully as you curve your back. Keep your breath even. Be aware of the spine from the very base to the top of the neck.

1. Kneel so that your hands rest directly below your shoulders, your knees below your hips. Hold your head in line with the spine. Check that your legs and arms are parallel to each other.

2. Inhale and arch your back. Expand your chest and let your neck curve backward. Keep your arms straight. Hold.

3. As you exhale, let your head lower toward your chest, and curve your back.

4. Continue in a flowing motion to curve and arch your back. Feel your back lengthening and loosening as you stretch.

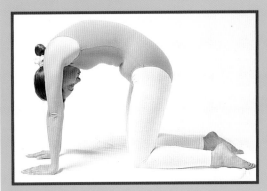

Step 2

Step 3

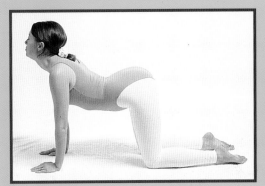

Cobra

As you practice this posture, visualize the graceful movements of a cobra. You will develop a supple spine if you practice this position regularly, and you will notice an improvement in your general well-being. It encourages fresh blood flow to the spine, the release of toxins, and the free flow of energy throughout the body.

1. Lie on your stomach and place your hands beneath your shoulders, palms flat on the floor, fingers facing forward, elbows close to your body. Legs and feet should be held together. Rest your forehead on the floor.

2. As you inhale, begin to raise your head from the floor. Once your head is a few inches from the floor, begin to raise your shoulders.

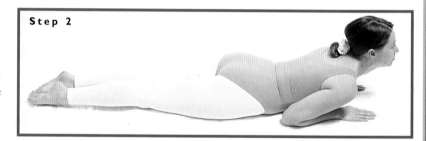

Step 2

3. Continue to lift your chest, your arms lengthening. Your hips remain on the floor. Stretch your chest forward. Your arms should still be bent at the elbow, your head facing forward.

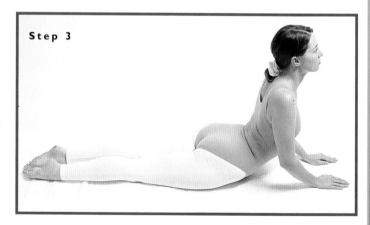

Step 3

4. Straighten your arms as much as you can without strain. Let your neck arch backward, and look toward the ceiling.

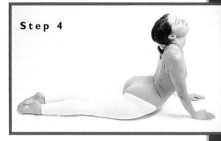

Step 4

5. As you exhale, lower your body, vertebrae by vertebrae, to the floor — chest first, then shoulders, and finally your forehead.

6. Rest in the Reversed Corpse pose.

Caution: Do not practice the Cobra if you have peptic ulcer, hyperthyroidism, hernia or have recently undergone any kind of abdominal surgery. Avoid during menstruation. Be careful if you have high blood pressure.

Corpse and Reversed Corpse

The Corpse and its reversed form are resting poses for the floor exercises. They are particularly suited to people who suffer neck and back problems. They elongate the spine after bending poses.

The Corpse

1. Lie on the floor on your back. Your feet should be a small distance apart, your arms resting comfortably at your sides. Face palms upwards.

2. Close your eyes. Let every muscle in your body soften and relax. Breathe deeply and slowly. Remain calm and still.

The Reversed Corpse

1. Lie on your stomach.

2. Part your legs a little, place arms by your sides, palms facing upwards.

3. Turn your head to one side. You may change the position of your head at any time if you feel the need.

Revive with Aromatherapy

The pleasant effects of scents can be more far-reaching than their appealing perfumes. Aromatherapy is the therapeutic use of scents in the form of essential oils.

Buying Essential Oils

Be careful when buying your essential oils that they are true essential oils and not those that have been adulterated or synthetically copied. If the label says "fragrant oil" or "aromatic oil" you are not buying a true essential oil. Buy your oils from a highly reputable supplier, and try to avoid oils that have been blended or diluted in carrier oils. The best carrier oils are nut or seed oils with a neutral aroma and labeling that says 100% pure, unrefined, and cold-pressed. Sweet almond oil and jojoba oils are both excellent carrier oils.

Essential oils are the aromatic essences extracted from plants, and each oil is made up of a number of different chemical constituents — it is these that give the oil its healing properties. Only a tiny amount is required to work its wonders.

There are many ways in which you can use essential oils. All methods ensure that the tiny molecules are absorbed rapidly into the bloodstream. They are then distributed to various organs and body systems, where they exert their therapeutic effect — calming your nerves if you are tense or anxious; helping you sleep if you suffer from insomnia; energizing you if you are fatigued. As well as influencing your emotions, essential oils can be of assistance in correcting many other bodily malfunctions, many of which drain your energy.

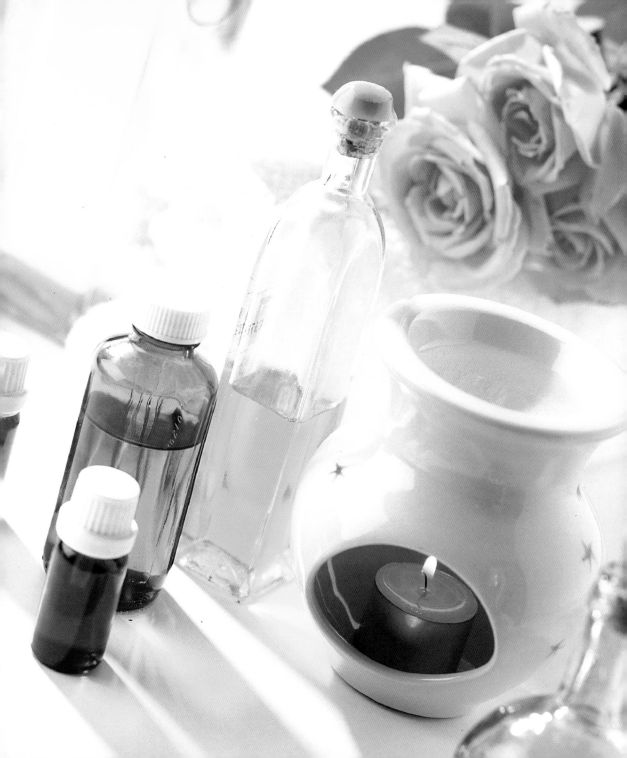

Methods for Using Essential Oils

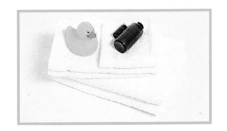

Vaporizers provide a favorite way to enjoy aromatherapy. Also called fragrancers, burners, aroma lamps, and diffusers, these containers (usually ceramic) have a bowl at the top and an opening for a candle at the bottom. Fill the bowl with hot water and add the essential oils. The candle keeps the water heated, releasing the fragrance into the atmosphere. Use 5 or 6 drops of essential oil. Take care not to let the water evaporate completely, as the oils will leave a sticky residue in the bowl.

Baths are a wonderfully relaxing way to enjoy aromatherapy. Try to lie in the bath for 20–30 minutes to allow the oils time to penetrate the skin. If you take your bath in the morning, the water should not be too hot. After the bath, stand under cool water to invigorate your skin and nervous system, and you will be energized for the day. If your bath is in the evening, for relaxation and to help you sleep, have the water as hot as you can. The heat will also create a vapor which you will inhale as you soak. Fill the bath with water, then add 6–12 drops of essential oil, swilling the water vigorously to ensure the oils are well dispersed.

Showers are sometimes more practical than baths because of time limitations. Sprinkle 2–3 drops onto a damp cloth and rub over the body while under the shower.

Candles and soaps impregnated with essential oils are commercially available, as are special-purpose combinations of essential oils.

Massage is a very comforting way to use essential oils. Aromatherapy massage can be relaxing, invigorating, or uplifting, depending on the oil chosen and the massage technique used. Measure 2 oz (50 ml) base carrier oil — sweet almond oil is a good one — into a glass bowl or bottle, add 10–25 drops of essential oils, and blend. Do not make up more than a week's supply of blended oils. Store your massage blend in a well-sealed, dark glass bottle in a cool dark place, and shake the bottle well before use. If you prefer to make a fresh mixture for each massage, the usual proportion is 2–3 drops of essential oil to 1 teaspoon (5 ml) carrier oil.

Compresses are soothing if you have a headache caused by tension and stress. Fill a bowl with ice cold water, add 6–10 drops of essential oil, and disperse through the water. Place a cloth in the water, then wring it out. Place on the forehead and temples for about 20 minutes. A soothing oil combination is 4 drops of lavender, 2 drops of orange, and 2 drops of chamomile.

Footbaths are wonderful for refreshing the feet, especially after a hard day's work or physical exercise. Add 4–8 drops of essential oil to a bowl of warm to hot water. Soak your feet for about 15 minutes.

A way of enjoying essential oils throughout the day, wherever you happen to be, is by sprinkling a drop of your chosen essential oil onto a tissue or handkerchief, so you can breathe in the vapors whenever you feel like it.

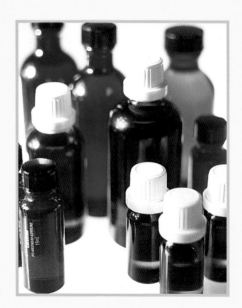

The Oils: What They Do, and How to Use Them

Oils can be used separately or in combination, though it is not a good idea to use more than 3 together. Not everyone likes, or responds to, the scents of all oils. Trust your own instinct as to the oil that will best suit you; for instance, if, when you smell the oil, you not only like the scent, but find yourself being uplifted, then that oil will work well in uplifting your mood.

To generate energy

Take a bath with 2 drops rosemary and 2 drops basil oil. You can also sprinkle 2 drops rosemary oil onto a tissue and inhale it throughout the day. Avoid these oils before bedtime as they are stimulating. Other oils which will increase your energy levels are orange, bergamot, lemongrass, juniper, rose, and peppermint.

To help you relax

A full body massage given to you by your partner or a friend will dispel all tensions. Oils that are good for relaxation are lavender, orange, rose, frankincense, vetiver, geranium, and patchouli.

Oils for Energy

- Basil
- Bergamot
- Juniper
- Lemongrass
- Orange
- Peppermint
- Rose
- Rosemary

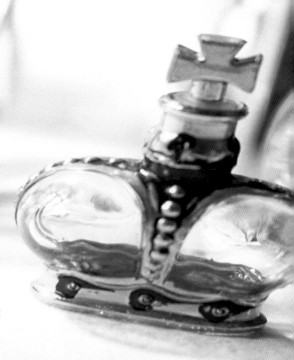

To help you sleep

The oils that help insomnia and restlessness have a sedative effect. Chamomile, orange, ylang ylang, geranium, lavender, rosewood, frankincense, and neroli are all good sedating oils. Soak in a bath, and add to a vaporizer near your bed.

To lift your mood

Oils that lift the mood without sedating are good for depression causing fatigue and lethargy. If you need to be uplifted, as well as comforted, massage with oils is a good idea. Make a mixture of 2 drops each of chamomile, geranium, and lavender oil in 3 teaspoons base carrier oil, and ask someone to massage you, or massage yourself (see COMING ALIVE WITH MASSAGE pages 54–59). Or use these oils, minus the carrier oil, in a bath. Other oils which are good for depression are orange, rose, and ylang ylang.

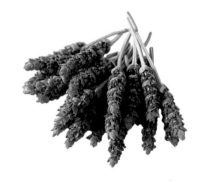

Come Alive with Massage

Tension-free muscles are needed for a relaxed state
of being, which is essential for high energy levels.

Begin a massage session by setting the scene — you can play relaxing music in the background or light some candles. A vaporizer, using a favorite essential oil, will also make the experience a pleasurable one.

If you don't have a massage partner on hand, indulge in some self-massage. This is a great way to loosen stiff muscles when you first wake up in the morning, after a hard day at the office, or those times when you require increased energy most. Before you begin, close your eyes and breathe deeply a few times. Keep your mind clear and your muscles relaxed.

The following sequences are for self-massage, but can be easily adapted for use by a partner.

Abdomen and chest

1. Lie on the floor with a pillow or rolled towel supporting your head. With one hand over the other, create circular movements in a clockwise direction over your abdomen.
2. Using your thumb and index finger, take some skin and give it a gentle pinch. Do this over your entire abdominal area, including your waist.
3. To stimulate your internal organs, massage over the large intestine. The movement should be done deeply and firmly. Draw the fingers of your right hand up from the groin area to the rib cage. Push across your abdomen to the left side, then, with the heel of your left hand, stroke down from the rib cage to the groin.
4. Gently massage your breastbone with the fingertips of both hands, using small circular movements.

5. Working slowly and carefully, and gradually increasing pressure as you feel the muscle tissue relaxing beneath your fingers, expand the area being massaged to the chest muscles and under the collarbone on both sides of your body, working toward the shoulders.

Neck and shoulders

1. To relax your neck muscles, use the palm and fingers of your left hand to stroke from the base of your scalp down the right side to your collarbone. Using the palm and fingers of your right hand, stroke from the base of your scalp down the left side to your collarbone.
2. Bring your left hand across your body to your right shoulder and knead the area by picking up flesh between your fingers, squeezing, then releasing.
3. Continue kneading all the way down the arm to the wrist, and then back up again.
4. When you reach your shoulder area again, work into it more deeply, with fingertips frictions (small circular movements). You can also use the heel of your hand. Increase the pressure as you feel the muscle tissue relaxing beneath your fingers.
5. Repeat steps 2–4 using the right hand on the left side of your body.

Scalp

1. Using the fingertips of both hands, move to the base of your skull. Start just behind the ears and work in small, deep, circular movements along the base of your skull to the middle of your neck. Work gradually, increasing pressure, until the knot has been smoothed away. If the knot is too tight, it is best to work on it in stages, over time.
2. With the same circular movements, working anticlockwise with the left hand, and clockwise with the right, move down the sides of your spine from the base of your skull to the shoulder blades.
3. To finish off, gently massage your entire scalp, using all your fingers in small circular movements. Feel the skin move under your fingertips. Then, using the same light movements, cover the back of the neck and the shoulders, and back up again over the scalp. Run the fingers of both hand through your hair from the front hairline, across the scalp, to the base of your neck.

Feet and Legs

People who are on their feet all day, or those who suffer from aching legs and feet, will find the following massage a true blessing. Begin by soaking your feet in warm water scented with your favorite essential oils — your feet should be clean when massaged. The following sequence can easily be adapted for two people. Feet can be ticklish so begin with firm pressure.

1. Sit on the floor with one leg extended. Bend the other leg and take hold of your foot. Stroke the sole of the foot with one hand.
2. Using your thumbs, make small penetrating circles over the entire sole, gradually increasing the pressure.
3. Squeeze your whole foot using both hands.
4. Extend your leg, keeping your knee bent, and fold the other one beneath your thigh. With both hands, reach down to your foot and, in one long, smooth movement, stroke up the front of your leg over the shin, the knee, and the thigh.
5. Repeat, but this time stroke up the back of the leg.
6. With your hands side by side, thumbs touching, apply long, even strokes with firm pressure from the foot to the knee, concentrating on the calf muscle.
7. Move up to the thigh and repeat the movement, pulling from knee to groin.
8. Knead the thigh area well. Work the outside of the muscle mass using thumb and fingers, alternately squeezing flesh then releasing it.
9. Repeat entire process to your other leg.

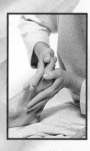

Hands and Arms

Whether you are receiving a massage or working on yourself, massage of the hands can be very reassuring and satisfying. Be dictated by your feelings, and create your own movements, your own massage style. Work on the palms, the backs of hands, the wrists, and each of the fingers.

1. Take your right hand and, beginning at the left wrist, stroke up the outside of the arm to the shoulder and back down the other side to the hand.
2. Knead all the way up the arm from the wrist to the shoulder, then back down the other side.
3. Take your left hand and, beginning at the right wrist, stroke up the outside of the arm to the shoulder and back down the other side to the hand.
4. Knead all the way up the arm from the wrist to the shoulder, then back down the other side.
5. Take your right hand and rub the palm with your left thumb. Stroke the upper surface of your right hand with the fingertips of your left hand. Gently rotate the wrist of your right hand.
6. With your left hand, take hold of each finger, in turn, of your right hand. Rotate each finger and, very gently, pull it away from the hand.
7. Take your left hand and rub the palm with your right thumb. Stroke the upper surface of your left hand with the fingertips of your right hand. Gently rotate the wrist of your left hand.
8. With your right hand, take hold of each finger, in turn, of your left hand. Rotate each finger and, very gently, pull it away from the hand.
9. With your left hand, gently stroke from your right shoulder down the arm to the hand, gliding off the fingers.
10. With your right hand, gently stroke from your left shoulder, down the arm to the hand, gliding off the fingers.

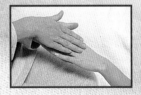

A Quick Reviving Massage

This massage requires two people and takes from 5 to 10 minutes to do. It can be performed at work, at home, anywhere, and will give hours of relief from stress and tension. It is best to have your partner sit astride a chair, with arms folded and head resting on the arms. A cushion or pillow can add extra comfort.

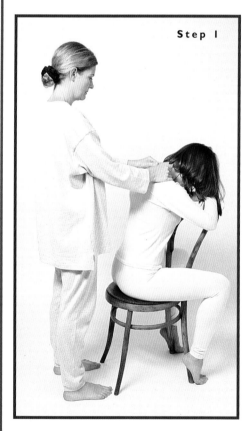

Step 1

1. Start at the shoulders using kneading movements. Squeeze and release with both hands at the same time. Work the whole shoulder area and then continue down the upper arms.

2. Using small, deep friction movements (small circular movements) with the pads of your thumbs, work the shoulder area and base of the neck.

3. Place one thumb on each side of the base of the neck and apply firm pressure — hold your thumbs still and use your body weight for strength. Move your thumbs down the spine a little, then reapply pressure. Continue with thumb pressures down each side of the spine until you are parallel with the end of the shoulder blade.

4. With the same movement, work along the inside edge of the shoulder blade, moving upward toward the top of the shoulder.

5. Place the palm of one hand on your partner's forehead for support, and knead the base of the neck with the other hand.

6. Continue kneading up the neck to the base of the skull.

7. Using the pads of your fingers, create circular friction movements over the whole scalp area.

8. Return to the shoulders and apply gentle flicking movements to the whole upper back. Your hands should be relaxed, with palms facing one another, and the wrists should be soft. Create a light, fast, bouncy movement using the little finger edge of the hands. Be careful to avoid bony areas. This movement will help invigorate your partner.

9. With closed fists, gently press in with knuckles each side of the spine from the base of the neck to below the shoulder blades. Soothe the area with more kneading to the shoulders and down the arms.

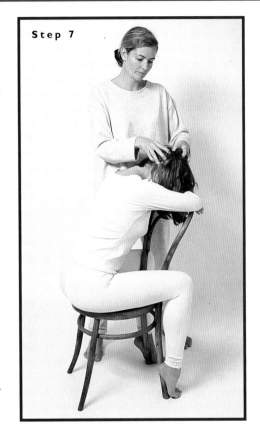

Step 7

10. Conclude the massage with light stroking over the whole area.

Your partner or friend will be reinvigorated and full of energy after this massage, their stress no more than a memory.

The Power of Crystals

Great powers have been attributed to crystals since humans first walked the earth. At certain times through history, crystals were believed to be a great source of energy and to have mystical powers as well as the ability to heal the body — some belief systems considered them living entities.

Many people today believe all these things to be true of crystals. When you see them displayed in a crystal store, you will perhaps understand why, because their beauty is remarkable. Take your time looking at the stones, and if one in particular draws your attention, hold it in your hands. If strong feelings are generated within you, it means it is likely to be of benefit to you in some way.

The crystals listed below are believed to have properties that could help increase your energy levels.

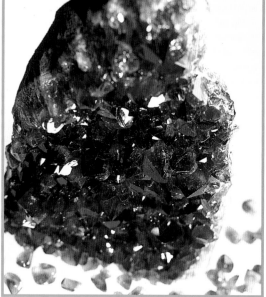

Amethyst

This stone is both stimulating and calming. It helps relieve the effects of stress and is recommended for those who suffer from insomnia or restless sleep, since it induces a state of tranquillity. The influence of amethyst assists the holder overcome addictive behavior and negative beliefs.

Clear Quartz

When held in the hand, clear quartz has been shown, through the use of Kirlian photography, to increase the amount of energy in the body. It clears congestion and blockages of energy channels, and relieves fatigue and lethargy. This stone enhances emotional energy, and encourages a positive and purposeful outlook on life.

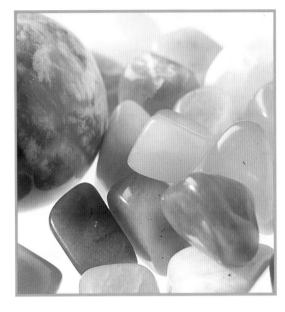

Yellow Fluorite

Fluorite helps give us a sense of inner peace; it also enhances mental clarity, especially during mentally stressful situations. Yellow fluorite assists the rejuvenation of body cells, and will help the liver eliminate fat and toxins from the body. An ideal choice for someone working under mental pressure.

Jade

This stone is beneficial to the kidneys, digestive system, and the heart. Jade is found in several colors, each of which has a different influence. Blue jade is a calming stone. Red jade is powerful and stimulating, and can help release tensions. Yellow jade improves a sluggish digestive system and tones the liver, thereby increasing physical energy.

Labradorite

Labradorite is believed to increase the efficiency of the body's metabolism. It improves the functioning of the digestive system, and the elimination of toxins and waste products from the body. Labradorite encourages us to let go of old behavior patterns and bad habits, anxieties, and negative beliefs. It is also said to motivate us to achieve our goals.

Smoky Quartz

Smoky quartz assists the body's digestive system by improving absorption of vital nutrients and helping in the elimination of wastes. It is also useful in calming anxieties and hyperactivity. As well, the influence of this stone can help lift bad moods and mild depression. It is believed to give the holder courage to try again.

Tiger's Eye

Tiger's eye balances the energy of the body, and helps the elimination of toxins. It encourages the holder to have a positive outlook, self-confidence, and optimism. Tiger's eye balances the emotions and gently awakens the intuition, making it an ideal stone for those who are developing an interest in spiritual matters.

Turquoise

Turquoise helps in the recovery from illness, especially where new tissue is being regenerated. It is a cooling, soothing stone, and helps the holder express emotions. It also encourages creative expression. Turquoise is effective during traumatic events, as it helps the holder stay calm and balanced, thus more able to deal with matters.

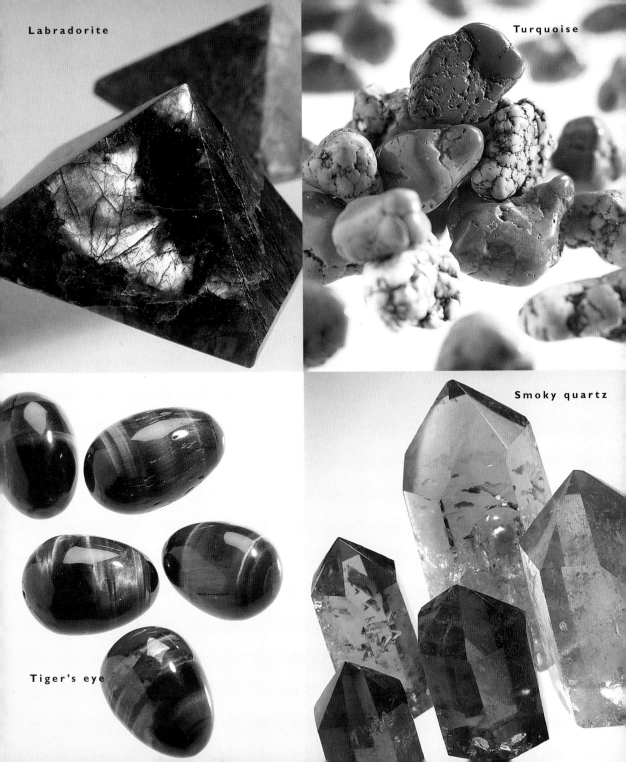

Labradorite

Turquoise

Smoky quartz

Tiger's eye

Color Energies

Color can suggest enthusiasm, gentleness, adventure, energy, love. It can also signal power, ruthlessness, coldness, control. But whatever the message conveyed, life in all its aspects is represented in the living vibration of color.

Color radiates energy. Color is all around us, in nature, in our clothing, our houses, our cars, everywhere. We consider color in relation to choosing a new car, buying a new article of clothing, or redecorating the home. Then the consideration is often one of what color in is fashion, not "How does it make me feel?"

Yet we all have colors we love and colors we detest. When we meet people we particularly like, we ask them their favorite color. In celebrity interviews, "What is your favorite color?" is a basic question. We feel a great affinity with people who share the same color tastes as our own. Despite the frequency with which color enters our conversations, we don't actually realize just how much it can affect our moods and vitality.

Imagine for a moment living in a world of varying tones of gray — how does that make you feel? Flat and depressed, no doubt. Gray radiates no energy, and our energy feels as though it is being absorbed into the grayness, with nothing coming back to replace that energy.

Wearing Color

The way we dress indicates to others how we see ourselves and how they should respond to us. Our choice of color depends on fashion and the colors that suit us, but sometimes our state of mind can also influence our choice of color. Overweight, shy, or insecure people frequently wear dark or drab colors because they do not wish to draw attention to themselves. In this, they are telling themselves they are unattractive, so they radiate feelings of inferiority and powerlessness. And the longer they wear these lifeless, drab colors, the more entrenched those feelings will become.

If you fall into this category, try wearing vibrant colors — even if it's only in the form of a scarf — and stand tall. How do you feel? Go out wearing these fabulous colors, and notice the difference in the way people respond to you. Positive, energetic colors lend you their energies.

The same principle can apply in reverse. If you are wound up with anxiety or tension, wearing calming greens and gentle blues could help you feel more relaxed.

Only you know, in the end, how each color makes you feel, therefore, what colors suit you best. Color can enhance your moods or alter them. Learn what effects various colors have on your moods. And remember, a splash of scarlet, whether it be in your lipstick or scarf, tie or handkerchief, may be all you need to give you that extra boost.

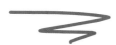

Some Colors and Their Effects

Yellow is the nearest color to light. It shines outward. It radiates energy, and does not wish to be confined. Yellow is the color of the sun. The sun gives life and warmth to all living things. The sun's light radiates through the universe. Yellow is the color of liveliness, happiness, gentleness, and stimulation. However, yellow must be kept pure in its color. A "dirtying" of the color prevents its energy from shining forth, and so creates a dulling, depressing effect on our moods.

Red is the color of activity and celebration — red finds it difficult to stay still, to be stagnant. See, in your mind's eye, a black leather couch. It's elegant, it is stillness itself. Now, put a red cushion on it. What happens to the still black color? It is suddenly vivid. There is now a sense of vibration, of movement, on that couch. Red is a color children love to play with. In their first paintings, they will use more red than any other color.

Green is the image of life; it is peaceful and soothing. Imagine a green field with some tall trees topped by green foliage of different hues - you may feel you could sit and look at the green field all day long. Now imagine some figures clothed in red on the field. What are they doing? Are they standing still like the trees? Or are they moving about — running, dancing, playing?

Blue is the color of the sky and of lakes and calm seas. In its paler hues, it is a calming color, and conveys lightness of spirit and a sense of freedom; however, it can be cold and oppressive if used in large amounts in its stronger tones.

Browns and beiges are the colors of fall or autumn. They can be soothing, especially if you have a strong personality or dramatic coloring. Whether you have used them in the color scheme of your home or as your basic color for dress, they can easily be dressed up with vivid scarves, handkerchiefs, or shirts.

Black is a color which radiates no energy in itself, but which makes other colors appear more vivid by its contrast. Like all colors, it can have a positive or negative effect, depending on how it's used. It can be depressing when the wearer's purpose is to hide. If the intention is to intimidate, black can be forceful, signaling power and control.

White radiates more energy than all other colors. However, it can be perceived as cold and intimidating. In other circumstances, white can radiate peace and harmony, especially when used with small amounts of other colors of a gentle or positive nature, like warm, pale blues or soft yellows.

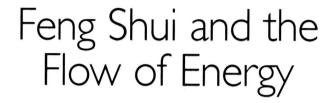

Feng Shui and the Flow of Energy

Good feng shui will improve your health and happiness,
and fill your environment with energy.

Feng shui (pronounced "foong swee" in Cantonese and "fong shwee" in Mandarin) is an ancient Chinese theory of design and placement. The basis of the theory is that you are affected by the way the life energy, the qi (chi), flows within and around your surroundings. You can improve the feng shui of your home or office simply by making alterations to your surroundings. This can be done by physically altering structures, like installing a skylight or window, or by moving furniture around. Changes can also be made, working on the level of altering your perceptions, with the use of "cures," such as wind chimes, bamboo flutes, fish tanks, plants, crystals, mirrors, or water.

The Front Door

Both people and positive qi will be attracted by a welcoming entrance:

- Always keep the front door in good repair
- Remove clutter or untidiness
- Make sure the lighting is good, and
- Keep a porch light on at night.

Feng shui means the flow of wind and water. The wind disperses the invisible life energy, the qi (chi), and the water contains it. The object of feng shui is to allow the qi energy to move around your home with ease, without getting trapped in corners or halted by obstructions. Qi flows more effectively along curving lines than straight lines. Angles and corners produce "secret arrows" of negative sha qi (shar chi) so need to be negated. This can be done by screening the offensive corner with potted plants, trees, wind chimes, or crystals.

Cures for Common Problems

Symmetry is important in all aspects of feng shui, including your home's decor. Whether you are choosing a piece of furniture, an ornament, or pot plant, ensure that its shape is balanced.

If you have an L-shaped room it is important to create two contained spaces, by using a screen, partition, or bookshelves.

The shape of the **furniture** should reflect the shape of the room. If you have a square room, use a square, round, or octagonal table. If the room is rectangular, a rectangular table is best. The placement of furniture should follow the protective "armchair" shape favored for the position of house and land in feng shui. This way, beneficial qi can enter, move around slowly, then return to nature. Where possible, place furniture against the four walls. Avoid placing chairs in a position that puts the occupier's back to a full length window or door because it will make him or her feel insecure.

Color can make a room seem larger or smaller, warmer or cooler; it can also make a room cheerful or depressing.

Indoor plants are useful for hiding sharp corners that generate "secret arrows" of sha qi.

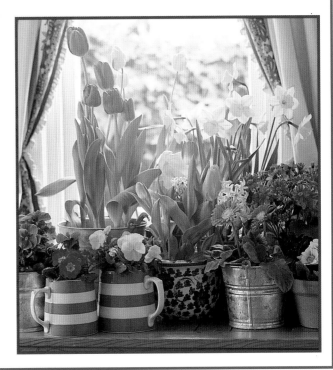

Install a **fish tank filled with goldfish** as their movement and color can help stimulate qi, which could boost your finances. The most auspicious numbers of goldfish are three, six, eight, or nine.

Symmetrical, faceted **crystals** hung in the center of a window will bring qi into a room.

Light represents energy and natural light is good feng shui. Overhead lighting can be harsh and oppressive. Table lamps create soft pools of light, which encourage relaxation. Candles add yang (male) qualities to a yin (female) area.

Mirrors can deflect negative sha qi and encourage positive sheng qi. Position a mirror where it can reflect a pleasant scene from outside, or in a windowless room like a bathroom.

When you hear the gentle singing of **wind chimes,** you know that stagnant qi is being activated. If you can see your back door from your front door, qi will run straight through, without having a chance to move around your home, bringing you prosperity and opportunity. Wind chimes hanging just inside the front door will help slow the qi down.

Water represents life and good fortune and brings positive energy. Moving water, like fountains and aquariums, can help stimulate qi — its effect is also calming. Ponds should be of natural shape, and their banks should be sloping.

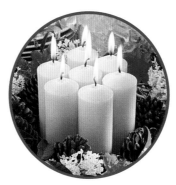

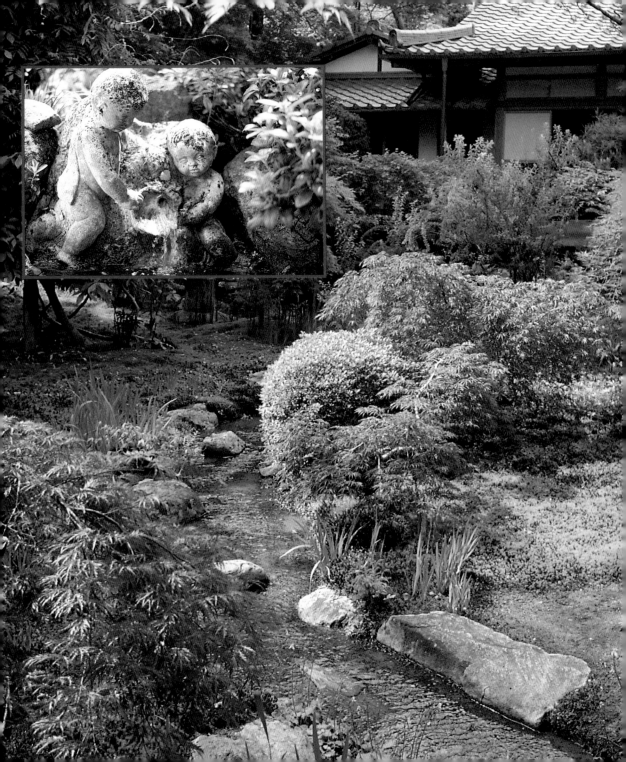

Revitalize Yourself with Nature

A bright bunch of flowers is cheerful and can be instantly uplifting.

Trees and plants emit not only oxygen, which is essential to our energy levels, but energy itself. While it is not necessary to go out and hug a tree (though it would do you no harm), it is essential for all of us to have some contact with nature on a regular basis, if not daily. Going for walks in a park or weekends in the wilderness are both great ways to revitalize your energy levels. But it is also a good idea to have some living plants in your home and office environment.

In Your Apartment or Office

If you have a balcony, you have room for a collection of potted plants. Pots come in all shapes and sizes, in different materials, different colors, and some are even decorated. There are

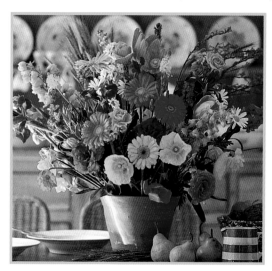

many plants that will suit your balcony in your climatic conditions. Your nearest garden center will advise you in your choice of plants. As you tend your plants, you will find yourself relating to them as living things, and you will find them a great source of peace.

If you do not have a balcony, but have light coming in through a window, you can place a pot plant either on the windowsill or on the floor. There are other plants that prefer low light conditions, such as African violets, a beautiful plant for which people frequently form an addiction.

In Your Backyard

If you already have a garden and tend it well, you are aware of the joy gardening brings, as well as the physical benefits you reap.

If you have never built a garden or know nothing about gardening, then it is never too late to learn. Even if you think you will hate it, try it — it will become one of the great joys of your life. Getting dirty is a great releaser of tensions. As well, you will have something beautiful to look at when you glance out of your windows.

You do not need a great deal of land — even the smallest space can support a garden. Garden beds do not have to be along the edges of straight paths or against fence lines. They can be in the middle of a lawn, they can be round, or of more creative shapes. Their shapes should flow in relation to other garden beds, paths, trees, and the house, and their edges should be curved.

Gardening usually becomes an addiction. Many people who have considered themselves uncreative have found they have a great feel for garden design. Like any other creative activity, follow your intuition.

Gardening is a wonderful exercise, a great soother of nerves, and a means of being in touch with yourself and in harmony with the natural world.

The Uplifting Effects of Music

Almost all people respond to music in some form or another. Music is used for fun, for releasing tension, for comfort, for getting away from yourself, and for uplifting the spirit. Music can also inspire you into action.

If you have trouble focusing or maintaining concentration when doing difficult mental work, music can help you. Recent studies have shown that students perform better in exams if they listen to classical music, especially Mozart, immediately prior to an exam — their IQs are actually increased for that period of time. The studies included a range of music. While rock music was not as effective as classical, it still rated better than no music at all.

Everyone should sing — ballads, rock, classical — and you don't need to know the words. It doesn't matter if you don't "have a voice," sing anyway. Singing uplifts the spirit, and is a great way to dispel negative emotions.

Dance away despondency and elevate your energy. Dance to rock music, to classical music; dance fast or slow, and make whatever movements you feel like at the time. Be creative in your movements, and feel yourself inside the music and as part of the music.

If you are intending to undertake some study or mental work, choose music from the *Music for Focusing* list opposite. If you need energizing or need to be inspired, choose music from the *Music for Inspiration and Energy* category. At the end of the day, while you are in your aroma bath or are unwinding, music from the *Music for Relaxation* category will best suit you.

Music for Focusing

Goldberg Variations by J.S. Bach (piano or harpsichord)
The Well-Tempered Clavier, Books I and II by J.S. Bach (piano or harpsichord)
Sonatas for Viola da Gamba and Keyboard by J.S. Bach (cello and piano or harpsichord)
Sonatas for Violin and Keyboard by J.S. Bach
Nisi Dominus, RV 608 by Vivaldi (countertenor and baroque orchestra)
Piano concertos nos. 20, 21, 23, 24 by Mozart) (piano and orchestra)
Waltzes by Chopin (piano solo)

Music for Inspiration and Energy

St Matthew Passion by J.S. Bach (choral work)
Magnificat in E flat major, BWV 243 by J.S. Bach (choral work)
The Four Seasons by Vivaldi (violin with stringed orchestra)
Pianos concertos nos. 20, 21, 23, 24 by Mozart (piano and orchestra)
Moonlight, *Pathetique*, *Appassionata*, *Walstein*, *Tempest* piano sonatas by Beethoven
Piano concertos nos. 1, 3, 4, 5 by Beethoven) piano and orchestra
Polonaises by Chopin (piano solo)

Music for Relaxation

Adagio in G minor by Albinoni (strings and organ)
Pastoral Symphony by Beethoven
Lieder by Schubert (for low voice or high, male or female)
The complete Nocturnes by Chopin (piano solo)
Panus Angelicus by Caesar Franck (voice)
Piano Quintet in A Op. 81 by Dvorak (piano and string quartet)
Vocalise by Rachmaninoff (soprano and orchestra)
Adagio for Strings by Samuel Barber
The Lark Ascending by Vaughan Williams (orchestral)

Quick Tips for Energy

To Combat Mental Fatigue

• Take three deep breaths in and out whenever you feel tired.
• Stretch and yawn — the louder the yawn the better.
• When you're feeling mental exhaustion at work, or for 5 minutes every hour, get up and pace around your office, or walk quickly or run up and down a flight of stairs. This will improve the flow of blood to your brain.
• Take a real lunch break. Organize workmates to go to the park for a regular, once-a-week picnic.
• Stop, rest and revive — short breaks will help prevent fatigue. A rest break need only take 30 seconds and consist of no more than a yawn and a stretch.
• Throw a tantrum! It's great for releasing mental or emotional tensions.

On Food

• First thing in the morning, a cup of lemongrass tea or a tea made from lemon-lime-lemongrass mixture will wake you up, as well as having a tonic effect on your liver. Dandelion tea is also good for the liver.
• For your morning coffee break, try stimulating rosehip tea or peppermint tea.
• Never go for more than 4 hours without something to eat. If you allow yourself to get too hungry, you will eat anything handy and sweet. Eat small quantities of high-fiber, low-fat food several times a day.
• Put variety into your diet — this will ensure you get all the right nutrients.
• Cut down on — better still, give up — pastries, pies, sugar, chocolate, and all fast foods. They give you an immediate boost, but half an hour later your energy is zapped!

For Exercise

• Work out at lunchtime. Even if it's for only a few minutes a day, do some exercise. Going for a walk — even pacing the floor — keeps blood circulating to the brain.
• Set yourself up so you have to get up to answer the phone or go to your filing cabinet.

For Feeling Great

• Before your shower, invigorate your body by brushing it with a soft, natural bristle brush or loofah. Begin from the toes and work your way up your body with long, firm strokes. Then, in long, firm strokes, brush your arms, starting at the wrists. Keep your brushing wrist loose.
• Sing in the shower and don't care what anyone thinks — it will definitely lift your mood. Wear something special today — a favorite shirt or your most colorful one, or something you keep only for the best occasions. Add a dab of your favorite scent.
• When you feel tired, overworked, or frazzled during the day, spray your face with a spritzer of 3–6 drops of essential oil to each 1 oz (30 ml) distilled, purified, spring, or mineral water. Oils to stimulate include lemon, orange, peppermint, bergamot, eucalyptus, and tea tree. Or you may prefer more soothing oils like chamomile, cypress, geranium, lavender, rosemary, or thyme. Sedating and relaxing oils include cedarwood, frankincense, jasmine, myrrh, neroli, patchouli, rose, sandalwood, and ylang ylang. You can mix 2 or 3 of these oils to suit your own taste.

Feeling great means being full of energy!

Index

Copyright © Lansdowne Publishing Pty Ltd

First published 1997
This edition published 1999

TIME-LIFE BOOKS IS A DIVISION OF TIME LIFE INC.

TIME LIFE CUSTOM PUBLISHING

Vice President and Publisher	Terry Newell
Associate Publisher	Teresa Hartnett
Vice president of Sales and Marketing	Neil Levin
Director of New Product Development	Quentin McAndrew
Director of Special Sales	Liz Ziehl
Project Manager	Christopher Register

TIME-LIFE is a trademark of Time Warner Inc. U.S.A.

ISBN 0 7835 5255 6

No data available upon application:
Librarian
Time-Life Books
2000 Duke Street
Alexandria, VA 22314

Printed in Singapore by Tien Wah Press (Pte) Ltd